DIY HOMEMADE HAND SANITIZERS

The Best Guide for Beginners to Make Your Natural Sanitizer for You and Your Family

Vanessa Rodriguez

Copyright & Disclaimer @Copyright 2020 by_____

All the content and graphics published in this e-book are the property of_____. The user of this e-book is prohibited to reuse, retain, copy, distribute or republish any contents or a part of contents of this e-book in any manner without written consent of the publisher.

Table of Contents

Chapter 1: Are homemade sanitizer alright for skin 1

Chapter 2: How to Properly Use Hand Sanitizer 3

Chapter 3: How handsantizers are useful? 12

Chapter 4: How to Clean and Disinfect Yourself, Your Home, and Your Stuff 17

Chapter 5: Kitchen surface freshner 20

Chapter 6: DIY Natural Toilet bowl Cleaner 26

Chapter 7: Natural floor cleaner disinfectant spray 51

Chapter 1: Are homemade sanitizer alright for skin

Hand sanitizer is taking off store retires in the U.S. as people and organizations stock up on provisions to ensure them against coronavirus disease.

General wellbeing specialists exhort that cleaning your hands with either cleanser and water, or a liquor based arrangement, is perhaps the most ideal approaches to stay away from contamination — the direction the general population seems, by all accounts, to be noticing. Buyer interest for hand sanitizers has taken off 1,400% as of late, as indicated by retail industry information. A few merchants are restricting the quantity of compartments clients can purchase per visit, while others are raising their costs in stores and on the web.

Fortunately, specialists have an attainable answer for customers who can't locate the individual disinfectant in stores: Make your own.

"Custom made hand sanitizers are similarly as successful as what you purchase as long as you utilize the correct level of liquor," CBS News benefactor Dr. David Agus told CBS MoneyWatch. "This is a decent method to get around individuals cost gouging for Purell."

Do-it-without anyone else's help sanitizers must contain at any rate 60% liquor, by volume, to work, Dr. Agus said. Isopropyl liquor (otherwise called scouring liquor) or ethanol are both appropriate assortments, specialists told CBS MoneyWatch. Different specialists prescribe utilizing in any event 90% liquor to guarantee the hand-made sanitizer is sufficient and to stay away from any danger of weakening the compound if different fixings are included, for example, aloe vera.

"On the off chance that you make it well, it's about as compelling as utilizing cleanser and water," said Dr. Stephen Morse, a teacher of the study of disease transmission at Columbia University in New York. "We realize it works — simply ensure it has enough liquor in it."

Including aloe vera will make it simpler to apply to the skin and include thickness. What's more, mixing in a couple of drops of a basic oil, for example, lavender, will give the blend a satisfying scent — so clients don't possess an aroma like scouring liquor around the home or office.

Chapter 2: How to Properly Use Hand Sanitizer

At the point when sanitizers initially came out, there was little research demonstrating what they did and didn't do, yet that has changed. More research should be done, however, researchers are learning all the more constantly.

The dynamic fixing close by sanitizers is isopropyl liquor (scouring liquor), a comparable type of liquor (ethanol or n-propanol), or a blend of them. Alcohols have for some time been known to kill microorganisms by dissolving their defensive external layer of proteins and disturbing their metabolism.

As per the CDC, inquire about shows that hand sanitizer eliminates germs as adequately as washing your hands with cleanser and water—except if your hands are noticeably grimy or oily. They additionally don't evacuate possibly destructive chemicals.

Hand sanitizers likewise don't murder some normal germs cleanser and water do kill, for example,

Cryptosporidium

Clostridium difficile

Norovirus

Microbes and Virus Protection

The U.S. Nourishment and Drug Administration (FDA) has made a legitimate move against some hand sanitizer organizations for making dubious cases against salmonella, e. Coli, Ebola, rotavirus, flu, and MRSA (methicillin-safe Staphylococcus aureus).

Simultaneously, however, examines are starting to recommend that liquor based hand sanitizers might be viable at murdering a portion of these germs. (All things considered, the organizations that cause them to still can't seem to pick up FDA endorsement for these utilizations, making any cases to this end illicit.)

For instance:

A recent report on emergency clinic borne contaminations shows sanitizers may help moderate the spread of MRSA and different diseases by giving a speedy, simple, and advantageous path for social insurance laborers to improve their hand hygiene.4

Research distributed in 2015 reasoned that liquor based sanitizers had the option to lessen the populaces of salmonella and E.coli.

Serious hand-sanitizer use in Japan in light of an influenza pandemic may have stopped term paces of norovirus.6

In an investigation on grade schools, hand sanitizers slice nonattendances because of sickness by 26% and diminished affirmed instances of ailment from the exceptionally infectious flu An infection by 52%. It was, be that as it may, less viable against the flu B virus.

A recent report on childcare focuses found a drop in days missed because of generally speaking disease when the inside presented hand sanitizers and instructed staff, youngsters, and guardians on their legitimate use.

In any case, it's essential to recall that not the entirety of the exploration is convincing. Truth be told, one investigation on long haul human services offices recommended that representatives' inclination for sanitizers over cleanser and water may have added to norovirus outbreaks.

Besides, the subtleties of a portion of these ends can be confounding. For instance, an examination distributed in 2019 noticed that an ethanol-based hand sanitizer decreased norovirus contamination hazard by 85% when there's transient contact with the infection. Be that as it may, under high-tainting conditions, for example, those you may discover on a voyage transport or in a drawn-out consideration office, the sanitizer offered no insurance whatsoever.

What to Look For

The CDC suggests sanitizers with at any rate 60% liquor content. Most items contain somewhere in the range of 60% and 95%, yet don't accept that the higher the rates are increasingly compelling. To work at top productivity, these items likewise need to contain some water.

A few items available cases to sterilize your hands yet contain too little liquor or no liquor by any stretch of the imagination. These items will probably not offer you satisfactory insurance.

Instructions to utilize it

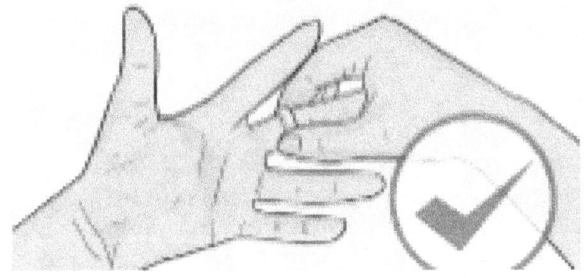

1. Away from the hands of all flotsam and jetsam and gems. Remove all rings and other adornments that might be covering the surfaces of your hands. On the off chance that conceivable, flush and evacuate all hints of obvious natural issue, for example, soil, oil, and nourishment all together for the hand sanitizer to be best.

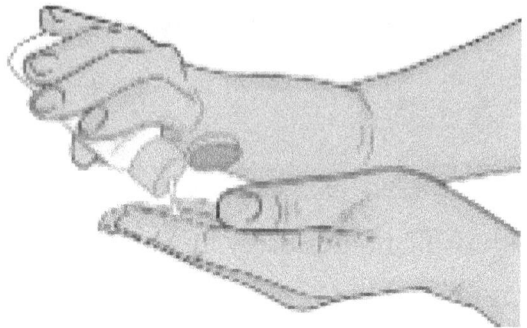

2. Spurt the hand sanitizer into the palm of one hand. Be liberal with the measure of sanitizer applied. At least, you should utilize a sum that is about the size of a U.S. quarter.

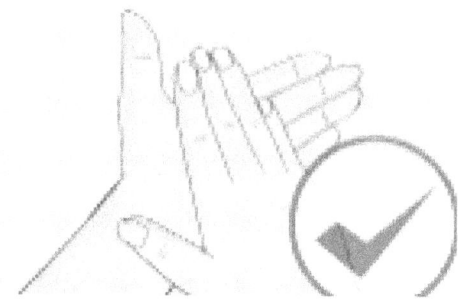

3. Rub your hands together delicately. Make certain to cover the surfaces of both of your hands, including fingers and around your fingertips and nails. You ought to likewise focus on the sanitizer around 2 inches (0.051 m) up every wrist.

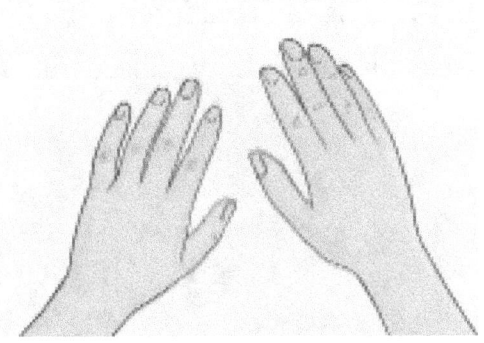

4. Let your hands get dry. After around 30 seconds of scouring, your skin ought to have ingested the sanitizer. If your hands are still somewhat wet, face your palms descending and let them dry noticeable all around until they are not, at this point wet.

Realizing When to Use Hand Sanitizer

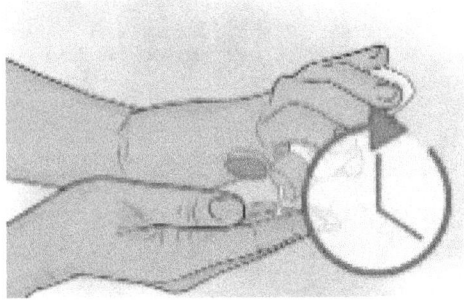

1. Use hand sanitizer intermittently for the day. Certain exercises or settings can present to a greater degree a hazard for the spread of diseases or ailments on the off chance that you have come into contact with creatures, individuals, or food. Consider what you have been contacting and who you have been

in contact with. Utilizing sanitizer intermittently during the day can help decrease the opportunity of becoming ill.

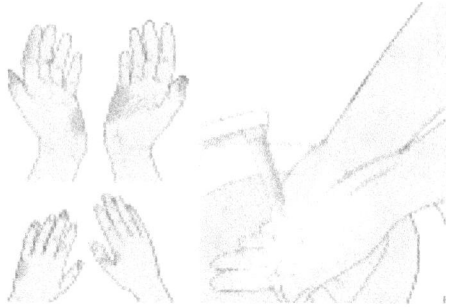

2. Flush your hands on the off chance that they are messy. Investigate the two sides of your hands and fingers to check whether there is any trash on them. Check whether there is any development gotten underneath your fingernails. Search for any open injuries, cuts or scratches. Hand sanitizer is best when applied to clean hands.

Because of its liquor content, hand sanitizer may disturb the injuries. This agony can be awkward, yet it is just impermanent.

3. Clean your hands with cleanser much of the time. The best method to expel or deactivate germs is to clean your hands with clean running water and cleanser. Notwithstanding, commonly it is beyond the realm of imagination to expect to find a restroom or sink right away. For this situation, hand sanitizer is

intended to be utilized as an advantageous choice to help decrease the spread of germs and the potential possibility of illness.

Hand sanitizers may not evacuate or deactivate destructive synthetics. On the off chance that you have been presented to any synthetic compounds or pesticides, you should wash the uncovered region with cleanser and water and talk with a specialist is fundamental.

Chapter 3: How handsantizers are useful?

How successful is hand sanitizer in forestalling sickness? The appropriate response may astonish you.

If you've visited a medication store recently, you most likely saw the void racks where hand sanitizers regularly sit.

With the coronavirus (COVID-19) flare-up, it's not amazing that numerous individuals are finding a way to remain safe, including loading up on purifying showers, gels, and cleansers. In any case, are hand sanitizers the best protection against microscopic organisms and infections like coronavirus and flu?

Organizations that advertise these items (which are here and there marked "antibacterial" or "antimicrobial") state yes. In any case, some customer advocates state no, contending that they aren't successful and can cause bacterial strains that oppose anti-toxins.

Incidentally, the best answer is to adopt a presence of mind strategy.

How valuable are hand sanitizers?

They're valuable in the emergency clinic, to help forestall the exchange of infections and microorganisms starting with one patient then onto the next by the medical clinic workforce. Past a clinic setting, it's extremely hard to show that hand purifying items are valuable.

Outside of the medical clinic, a great many people contract respiratory infections from direct contact with individuals who as of now have them, and hand sanitizers will do nothing in those conditions. Furthermore, they haven't been appeared to have more sterilizing power than simply washing your hands with cleanser and water.

Advantageous cleaning

The versatile hand sanitizers do have a job during the top respiratory infection season [roughly November to April] because they make it a lot simpler to clean your hands.

It's considerably more troublesome when you sniffle to wash your hands than it is to utilize a hand sanitizer, particularly when you are outside or in a vehicle. The hand sanitizers are substantially more advantageous, so they make it more probable that individuals will clean their hands, and that is better than not cleaning by any means.

As per the Centers for Disease Control (CDC), in any case, for hand sanitizer to be powerful it must be utilized effectively. That implies utilizing the correct sum (read the mark to perceive the amount you should utilize), and scouring it everywhere throughout the surfaces of two hands until your hands are dry. Try not to wipe your hands or wash them after applying.

Are all hand sanitizers made equivalent?

It's critical to ensure any hand sanitizer you do utilize contains in any event 60 percent liquor.

Studies have discovered that sanitizers with lower focuses or non-liquor based hand sanitizers are not as compelling at eliminating germs as those with 60 to 95 percent liquor.

Specifically, non-liquor based sanitizers may not work similarly well on various sorts of germs and could make a few germs create protection from the sanitizer.

Are hand sanitizers and other antimicrobial items awful for you?

There is no proof that liquor based hand sanitizers and other antimicrobial items are unsafe.

They could hypothetically prompt antibacterial opposition. That is the explanation regularly used to contend against utilizing hand sanitizers. Be that as it may, that hasn't been demonstrated. In the emergency clinic, there hasn't been any proof of protection from liquor based hand sanitizers.

In any case, while there aren't any investigations demonstrating that hand sanitizers unquestionably represent a danger, there likewise isn't any proof that they make a superior showing of shielding you from unsafe microscopic organisms than a cleanser.

So while hand sanitizers have their place — in emergency clinics or when you can't get to a sink — washing with cleanser and warm water is quite often a superior decision

Chapter 4: How to Clean and Disinfect Yourself, Your Home, and Your Stuff

THERE'S SOMETHING DEEPLY disrupting about venturing out of the home-from-work fatigue of self-confinement into the strained, encompassing frenzy of shopping for food during a pandemic. Typical is a twofold sided coin now. At home, things feel hyperreal, and outside they feel completely strange—two stages expelled from the flashback scenes in a dystopian film. You may feel a strain between helping yourself and helping your locale. Everyday life during the novel coronavirus pandemic is tied in with muddling contrasts like these.

It may appear to be increasingly profitable to peruse our Coronavirus Gear and Supplies Guide and begin filling your washroom with canned products and basics, however, cleaning and disinfecting surfaces in your home can help bring down the odds you or a friend or family member will contract COVID-19 and lower the odds you may spread it to another person. Keeping your home (and self) sterilized helps everybody.

The Centers for Disease Control prescribes we as a whole find a way to clean and purify high-contact surfaces in our homes.

Beneath, we get off course of to what extent the infection may keep going on surfaces, which disinfectants may murder it, and the means you should take to keep clean.

To Keep Yourself Virus-Free

Wash Your Hands

You've heard it a million times at this point, and you'll hear it a million more, however, the most ideal approach to bring down your danger of contracting COVID-19 (or give it to another person) is to wash your hands after you hack, sniffle, contact your face, utilize the bathroom, or are going to leave one spot for another. You should wash your hands when you leave and come back from the supermarket, for example.

On the off chance that you can discover any, hand sanitizer is a quick cleaning strategy that does something amazing. Hand sanitizer is not a viable alternative for washing your hands with cleanser and water, however. Utilizing cleanser and water can likewise be somewhat simpler on your hands. It won't really slaughter all pathogens, yet on the off chance that you wash your hands appropriately, it'll wash them away. The World

Health Organization has point by point guidelines (which we've all found in image structure) on the best way to appropriately play out the 20-recycled wash.

It's additionally imperative to generously saturate your hands. Dry, split skin is at more serious hazard for a wide range of contaminations, so after you wash, apply a little lotion. It's pleasant! Most saturating creams have comparative fixings, beginning with water and glycerin, so the brand doesn't generally make a difference. (Here are some hand moisturizers on Amazon.) If your hands are additional dry, search for something dermatologist-suggested with an "escalated" name, as Eucerin Advanced Repair or Neutrogena Hydro Boost.

Chapter 5: Kitchen surface freshner

It's not simply surfaced that need normal cleaning in the kitchen: the air is regularly weighed down with scents and cooking oils that make it substantial and disagreeable.

Business deodorizers regularly just cover hidden scents with counterfeit aromas that aggravate things smell, as opposed to better.

Obviously, nothing beats opening the windows wide and giving new breeze access to the kitchen! In any case, the awful climate can make this an unreasonable arrangement on occasion. Here are a couple of strategies for making fresher air utilizing regular family and nursery fixings.

Flavors AND CITRUS

This current one's a characteristic during the Christmas season, yet it works throughout the entire winter – or on any dark, melancholy day.

Liven up stale and stuffy air by stewing entire flavors and citrus strips.

To an enormous pot of water, include 1/4 cup entire cloves, 4 entire nutmegs, 6 cinnamon sticks, and the strip of 2 lemons or one orange.

Heat just to the point of boiling, at that point lessen the warmth and stew for an hour or thereabouts, to fill the kitchen with a zesty sweet aroma.

The sweet-smelling fluid can likewise carry out twofold responsibility, so don't hurl it out! At the point when cool, strain into a shower container to spritz when your home needs a touch of refreshing.

HERBS AND FRUIT

This one utilizes same thought as above, however with lighter aromas

Heat an enormous pot of water to the point of boiling, and include your preferred natural product cut into quarters, or a few twigs of nursery new herbs – or make a mix of both for your own mark fragrance.

Decrease warmth and stew for 1-2 hours, and appreciate the smell. At the point when cool, strain through a fine work screen and into a shower bottle, to spritz when the air needs a little shot in the arm.

Herbs with woody stems, for example, rosemary, lavender, thyme, cove leaves, or even southernwood (a restorative herb that is indigenous to southern Europe) are ideal for this.

They're better ready to keep up their respectability and aroma for longer periods in stewing water than verdant ones, however, any herbs will give a dazzling scent. Two or three delicate tips from a pine or cedar tree can likewise be utilized as such.

Apples, citrus natural product, pears, and cranberries all give a light, new aroma too.

SALT AND BAKING SODA

This mix is especially valuable for cleaning channels and disposing of the scents that originate from them.

Empty 1 cup rock salt into the channel, at that point 1 cup preparing pop. Let the bubbling activity of the sodium bicarbonate and the intensity of salt do the extreme cleaning work.

Follow with a pot brimming with dissipating water to flush gunk and scents.

Flawless LEMONS

Lemons have wonderful cleaning properties, and sprucing up the spot is just one of them.

For an unadulterated lemon aroma that eats up substantial oil particles, waiting for fishy scents, and other cooking smells, cut 2 lemons into equal parts or quarters.

Line a heating sheet with foil and spot the lemon pieces on top, with some breathing room in the middle. At that point heat in a 250°F broiler for 1-2 hours.

Subsequent to killing the warmth, leave the lemons on the plate. Open the stove entryway, and permit their purifying scent to keep working until the broiler is totally cool.

BORAX FOR THE GARBAGE PAIL

Borax is another valuable family unit cleaner that functions admirably for retaining scents.

Freshen up your trash bucket once every month by including 1/4 cup borax and 2 quarts of heated water. Wash the water around to cover the inside of your bucket, at that point spill the water out.

Flip around the bucket to deplete, and permit to dry. When dry, sprinkle some borax on the base for proceeded with scent insurance, at that point put in a waste sack.

This is additionally useful for expelling smells from kitchen manure containers and diaper buckets.

THE NOSE KNOWS

A new aroma in the kitchen not just causes the space to feel clean, it's an incredible state of mind lifter too!

Attempt these in your own kitchen and investigation with a portion of your preferred fragrances from flavors, herbs.

Chapter 6: DIY Natural Toilet bowl Cleaner

Regular Cleaners for Toilets

As a matter of first importance, there are a few common fixings you can use to figure a handcrafted latrine bowl cleaner. Additionally, making your permits you the opportunity to utilize whichever fixings you feel is most secure for your family. At long last, the fixings are promptly accessible and extremely powerful.

White Vinegar

You're presumably exhausted from hearing all the promotion on green-living sites about how magnificent vinegar is for characteristic cleaning. Be that as it may, I can't quit praising its excitedly. Vinegar is a mellow corrosive. It sanitizes, takes out scents, and is very sheltered.

Borax

In opposition to off base data on certain sites, borax isn't a similar thing as boric corrosive (which is harmful). It is sodium tetraborate, and is just as lethal as normal table salt or preparing pop, in exceptionally LARGE sums. Borax is an extraordinary multi-reason cleaner that brightens, freshens up, and expels stains.

Lemon Juice or Citric Acid

Citrus extract, additionally found in lemon juice, ties to minerals in the can bowl making them simpler to wipe out. It might help decrease intense can recolors left by hard water.

Basic Oils

Unadulterated basic oils are the absolute best clear-cut advantages to use in DIY cleaners. A large number of these plant-based oils brag antibacterial, antiviral, and even antifungal properties. Tea tree oil has been concentrated more than some other basic oil and has been found to slaughter most types of microscopic organisms when added to cleaners at a 0.5% – 1.0% fixation. Other basic oils that have antibacterial properties, and are helpful in restroom cleaners are lavender, citrus oils, peppermint, rosemary, and eucalyptus, among others.

Heating Soda

Heating soft drinks are awesome as a custom made latrine bowl cleaner. In particular, it scours and freshens up a can bowl normally. Significantly, it doesn't have any germ-battling benefits. Be that as it may, it will help keep your bowl liberated from flotsam and jetsam, stains, and those terrible rings.

Handcrafted Toilet Cleaner Formulas

Take your pick from these characteristic, natively constructed can bowl cleaner plans that we use and love.

Tea Tree Toilet Bowl Scrub

This freshening up recipe uses the antibacterial properties of tea tree oil to eliminate germs in your latrine bowl and on can surfaces.

½ cup heating pop

1 cup refined white vinegar

½ teaspoon tea tree basic oil

Join vinegar and fundamental oil in a little shower bottle. Splash vinegar blend inside the bowl, and on the latrine seat, cover, and handle. Permit the cleaner to sit for a few minutes. Sprinkle heating soft drink inside the can bowl and clean within the bowl with a latrine brush. Utilize a spotless dry fabric to clear vinegar arrangement off seat, cover, and handle.

Hardcore Toilet Formula

This latrine bowl recipe can deal with terrible rings in your chest, or some other intense can cleaning. It leaves a shimmering bowl and wipes out stale latrine scents.

¾ cup borax

1 cup white vinegar

10 drops lavender fundamental oil

5 drops lemon fundamental oil

Consolidate all fixings in a bowl or spurt bottle. Wash water around within the can bowl with a can brush, or essentially flush to wet within the bowl. Empty the whole blend into the can bowl, and permit it to sit for a few hours or overnight.

Ensure relatives don't utilize the latrine during this time. Clean the bowl and flush the latrine to wash.

Apathetic Day Toilet Scrub

For simple latrine cleaning, keep a splash jug of vinegar and a shaker-top jug of heating soft drink in your washroom. At the point when toilets need cleaning, spritz altogether with vinegar and permit to sit for a few minutes. Sprinkle preparing soft drink inside the bowl, clean within the bowl, and flush can. To clean the outside surfaces simply splash with vinegar, let stand a couple of moments, and wipe clean.

Common Homemade Toilet Bowl Cleaner Recipes

You can embrace one of these simple plans for cleaning your toilets. Or then again, you can try different things with the regular fixings talked about in this article to make your equation.

It is safe to say that you are attempting to carry on with a more beneficial, progressively manageable way of life? Wiping out compound cleaners from your house is an incredible spot to begin. We challenge you to begin with a custom made can cleaner. At that point, do one DIY cleaner seven days until every one of your cleaners is regular and handcrafted.

Need assistance? We composed a book that strolls you through the creation of all your characteristic family unit cleaners. You can discover it here.

Sources

Hydrochloric Acid. National Center for Biotechnology Information. PubChem Compound Database; CID=313. Betsy holds a four-year college education in Psychology and a Master's qualification in Counseling, and for about 10 years functioned as a rudimentary advisor. In 2011 she left her guiding profession to seek after sound living. She cherishes utilizing DIY Natural as an approach to instruct individuals to rely upon themselves to feed their bodies and live more joyful more beneficial lives. Associate with Betsy on Facebook, Twitter, and her +Betsy Jabs Google profile.

Step by step instructions to Make Whipped Soap DIY56

Figure out How to Make Soft and Creamy Whipped Soap!

Today you will figure out how to make whipped cleanser. This is a 2-advance procedure that includes making glue and afterward stirring the glue into a cleanser. Appreciate!

Normal Garbage Disposal Cleaner Recipe132

A Natural Garbage Disposal Cleaner and Deodorizer

I as of late made this normal waste disposal cleaner and deodorizer formula to refresh my stinky waste disposal. It is all-common and it works extraordinarily!

Hey all, I utilized the dental replacement tablet cleaner strategy also. At some point, while I was making shower bombs, I eyeballed the fixings in dental replacement tabs. Preparing pop and citrus extract!

Brenda RussellAugust 1, 2018 at 7:35 am

Yes. Vinegar outwardly, heating soft drink within – trailed by a flush and afterward a wash of vinegar (apprehensive of causing a volcanic response!). Been doing this for a considerable length of time, and never missed the business synthetic concoctions. Obviously, with three children, I escaped tidying up the yellow puddles behind the latrine by causing them to do it. Even though Not Me got the fault!

I love utilizing vinegar and heating soft drinks for cleaning, however for toilets I use store brand dental replacement tabs. Simply drop one in and hold up a couple of moments at that point wash. There is something in particular about the blue or green shading and the effervescing that I like.

Salt (NaCl) is utilized (alongside sulfuric corrosive) in the creation of hydrochloric corrosive (HCl), however, it is unquestionably not something very similar. Hydrochloric corrosive is a solid corrosive with a pH of about

1. You can see progressively about the threats of hydrochloric corrosive on a Material Safety Data Sheet for it:

I've attempted each sort of common thing for toilets. Nothing takes a shot at rust stains except Bar Keepers Friend. We have some rust even with an iron channel and water conditioner. BKF disposes of ALL sorts of stains on my old white porcelain.

To what extent would I be able to keep the vinegar blend expiry date as it were

The vinegar blended in with fundamental oils will save for a long while. (It's difficult to give precise exp. dates with custom made recipes.) I would suggest putting away the arrangement in a dim cabinet so the fundamental oil isn't continually presented to light.

I am pondering about the impact of the borax or the heating pop and vinegar on my septic tank??? I just dumped the suggested compound treatment down there two evenings before keep up the septic tank. Would any of this check or meddle with the chemicals? Would you be able to give me a reference I can check? Much appreciated.

Extraordinary inquiry Rosemarie. Borax, preparing pop, and vinegar is generally improved for your tank than substance cleanersGreat question Rosemarie, much obliged. As we, for a long time, are utilizing the EM (Effective-Micro living being) items and we are searching for our septic tank also.

Remember additionally never to blend smelling salts in with chlorine blanch as the mix of the two makes harmful vapor in huge amounts.

Fascinating inquiry! I have no clue if this one would stand up in court, particularly since an enormous level of the nation is as yet utilizing synthetic cleaners.

I had a companion who utilized a pumice stone purchased from the nearby home improvement shop to clean off the can rings that had amassed. She needed to enclose her hand by a dishtowel to utilize it, however, dang it if it didn't work!

(I simply utilize preparing pop and a clean brush. I do not pumice stone in-your-face yet.)

I have bought your book and utilize this formula on my latrine that my 4 young men use-the can come out extraordinary! Much obliged to you for sharing this information. I'm extremely glad to now be cleaning my home without lethal synthetic substances!

I would be anxious about the possibility that the pop or borax would check the corrosive in the vinegar and make it ineffective. Should I stress?

Any metal hydroxide (like heating pop) kills corrosive, similar to vinegar. Possibly take a stab at utilizing them independently...?

Sprinkle the soft drink on, at that point splash on the vinegar. The response happens on the bowl giving overwhelming cleaning activity. No concerns.

This is great; thanks to such an extent!!!

A debt of gratitude is for the new 'formula'. I utilize my clothing cleanser, frothing handsoap and general chemicals, and simply made some dishwasher cleanser the previous evening. I will be evaluating your latrine bowl cleaner. In the article, you referenced utilizing rosemary oil, which I have close by. Was it proposed in light of its smell, or does it have sterilizing – and other – properties useful for cleaning germy surfaces? A debt of gratitude is for your arrangement on DIY chemicals. What a simple method to set aside a wad of cash!

Truly, I love rosemary for its sterilizing properties! The new smell is only a reward.

What do you use for cleaning and disinfecting the latrine surface?

A shower of vinegar followed by a splash of peroxide or in any request will sterilize.

About Matt and Betsy

About Matt and Betsy

Matt and Betsy are enthusiastic about living normally and building a similarly invested network concentrated on the economical way of life.

DIY Natural is tied in with rediscovering the conventional benefit of doing things yourself, doing them normally, and getting a charge out of the advantages.

How to Clean Wood Furniture

You residue and sparkle your wood furniture routinely, yet after some time those finishes and residue consolidate to leave a dim film on tables, seats and retires. To keep your furniture putting its best self forward, you have to do an intermittent profound cleaning. Here are the means by which to clean wood furniture without harming its completion.

Residue the furniture to expel surface earth. Presently you're prepared to expel light ruining. Start with the gentlest cleaner and climb to more grounded ones varying. Take a stab at blending a powerless arrangement of water and dishwashing cleanser. Dunk a delicate fabric in the arrangement, wring it out and wipe the whole piece. You need a sodden material, not a wet one. Try not to soak the wood, and wash your material frequently. Take a second, clean material, and dry the piece completely.

Here's the manner by which to clean wood furniture that is recolored or has different issues.

Expel Old Polish

Realizing how to clean old wood furniture that has decades' old development of finish will assist you with renewing a collectible.

Steep two tea packs in bubbling water. Let the tea cool to room temperature, take a delicate fabric, wring it out in the tea until it's soggy and wash the wood. The tannic corrosive from the tea is superb for looking after wood. You'll be amazed at how the wood will sparkle.

Expel Water Stains

Here's the manner by which to expel water rings from wood where somebody has put a hot or cold beverage straightforwardly on a table. Put a spotlight on some non-gel toothpaste and rub with a delicate material till the stain is lifted. For obstinate stains, blend equivalent amounts of heating pop and toothpaste. Wipe the toothpaste off with a spotless sodden material and dry completely.

Eradicate Difficult Marks

To evacuate an ink mark, blend 1 tablespoon of heating pop and 1 teaspoon of water into a flimsy glue. Apply to the stain and rub tenderly with a delicate fabric until the stain vanishes. Wipe the toothpaste off with a spotless moist material and dry completely.

When your furniture is spotless, wipe a layer of wood finish on it to save the completion and include sparkle. You can utilize economically arranged lemon oil. You can likewise make a straightforward clean by blending 1 cup of olive oil in with 1/4 cup white vinegar. Pour it on a delicate material and work it into the wood, cleaning with the grain. Buff till sparkly. Realizing how to clean wood furniture will assist you with keeping your assets looking exquisite, longer. You residue and sparkle your wood furniture consistently, however after some time those finishes and residue consolidate to leave a dim film on tables, seats and retires. To keep your furniture putting its best self forward, you have to do an intermittent profound cleaning. Here's the way to clean wood furniture without harming its completion.

Residue the furniture to evacuate surface earth. Presently you're prepared to evacuate light ruining. Start with the gentlest cleaner and climb to more grounded ones varying. Take a stab at blending a frail arrangement of water and dishwashing cleanser. Dunk a delicate fabric in the arrangement, wring it out and wipe the whole piece. You need a sodden fabric, not a wet one. Try not to immerse the wood, and flush your material regularly. Take a second, clean material, and dry the piece altogether.

Here's the way to clean wood furniture that is recolored or has different issues.

Evacuate Old Polish

Realizing how to clean old wood furniture that has decades' old development of finish will assist you with reviving a collectible. Steep two tea sacks in bubbling water. Let the tea cool to room temperature, take a delicate fabric, wring it out in the tea until it's clammy and wash the wood. The tannic corrosive from the tea is brilliant for looking after wood. You'll be amazed at how the wood will sparkle.

Expel Water Stains

Here are the means by which to expel water rings from wood where somebody has put a hot or cold beverage legitimately on a table. Put a spotlight on some non-gel toothpaste and rub with a delicate fabric till the stain is lifted. For obstinate stains, blend equivalent amounts of preparing pop and toothpaste. Wipe the toothpaste off with perfect soggy material and dry completely.

Eradicate Difficult Marks

To evacuate an ink mark, blend 1 tablespoon of preparing pop and 1 teaspoon of water into a slim glue. Apply to the stain and rub tenderly with a delicate fabric until the stain vanishes. Wipe the toothpaste off with a spotless sodden fabric and dry completely.

When your furniture is perfect, wipe a layer of wood finish on it to safeguard the completion and include sparkle. You can utilize industrially arranged lemon oil. You can likewise make a basic clean by blending 1 cup of olive oil in with 1/4 cup white vinegar. Pour it on a delicate material and work it into the wood, cleaning with the grain. Buff till sparkly. Realizing how to clean wood furniture will assist you with keeping your assets looking exquisite, longer.

How to deep clean a garbage disposal

You residue and sparkle your wood furniture normally, however after some time those finishes and residue join to leave a dim film on tables, seats, and retires. To keep your furniture putting its best self forward, you have to do an intermittent profound cleaning. Here's the way to clean wood furniture without harming its completion.

Residue the furniture to expel surface soil. Presently you're prepared to expel light ruining. Start with the gentlest cleaner and climb to more grounded ones varying. Take a stab at blending a feeble arrangement of water and dishwashing cleanser. Dunk a delicate fabric in the arrangement, wring it out and wipe the whole piece. You need a sodden material, not a wet one. Try not to soak the wood, and flush your fabric regularly. Take a second, clean fabric, and dry the piece altogether.

Here are how to clean wood furniture that is recolored or has different issues.

Evacuate Old Polish

Realizing how to clean old wood furniture that has decades' old development of finish will assist you with reviving a collectible. Steep two tea packs in bubbling water. Let the tea cool to room temperature, take a delicate material, wring it out in the tea until it's clammy and wash the wood. The tannic corrosive from the tea is magnificent for looking after wood. You'll be astonished at how the wood will sparkle.

Evacuate Water Stains

Here's the way to expel water rings from wood where somebody has put a hot or cold beverage straightforwardly on a table. Put a spotlight on some non-gel toothpaste and rub with a delicate material till the stain is lifted. For obstinate stains, blend a balance of preparing pop and toothpaste. Wipe the toothpaste off with perfect sodden material and dry altogether.

Delete Difficult Marks

To expel an ink mark, blend 1 tablespoon of heating pop and 1 teaspoon of water into a meager glue. Apply to the stain and rub tenderly with a delicate material until the stain vanishes. Wipe the toothpaste off with a perfect sodden fabric and dry altogether.

When your furniture is perfect, wipe a layer of wood finish on it to safeguard the completion and include sparkle. You can utilize financially arranged lemon oil. You can likewise make a basic clean by blending 1 cup of olive oil in with 1/4 cup white vinegar. Pour it on a delicate fabric and work it into the wood, cleaning with the grain. Buff till sparkling. Realizing how to clean wood furniture will assist you with keeping your assets looking stunning, longer. You residue and sparkle your wood furniture routinely, however after some time those finishes and residue consolidate to leave a dull film on tables, seats, and retires. To keep your furniture putting its best self forward, you have to do an occasional profound cleaning. Here's how to clean wood furniture without harming its completion.

Residue the furniture to evacuate surface earth. Presently you're prepared to evacuate light dirtying. Start with the gentlest cleaner and climb to more grounded ones varying. Take a stab at blending a frail arrangement of water and dishwashing cleanser. Plunge a delicate material in the arrangement, wring it out and wipe the whole piece. You need a soggy material, not a wet one. Try not to immerse the wood, and wash your material regularly. Take a second, clean material, and dry the piece completely.

Here's the way to clean wood furniture that is recolored or has different issues.

Evacuate Old Polish

Realizing how to clean old wood furniture that has decades' old development of finish will assist you with reviving a collectible. Steep two tea packs in bubbling water. Let the tea cool to room temperature, take a delicate material, wring it out in the tea until it's clammy and wash the wood. The tannic corrosive from the tea is great for looking after wood. You'll be shocked at how the wood will sparkle.

Evacuate Water Stains

Here are how to expel water rings from wood where somebody has put a hot or cold beverage straightforwardly on a table. Put a spotlight on some non-gel toothpaste and rub with a delicate fabric till the stain is lifted. For difficult stains, blend equivalent amounts of heating pop and toothpaste. Wipe the toothpaste off with a perfect soggy fabric and dry completely.

Eradicate Difficult Marks

To evacuate an ink mark, blend 1 tablespoon of heating pop and 1 teaspoon of water into a meager glue. Apply to the stain and rub delicately with a delicate fabric until the stain vanishes. Wipe the toothpaste off with perfect sodden material and dry altogether.

When your furniture is perfect, wipe a layer of wood finish on it to save the completion and include sparkle. You can utilize financially arranged lemon oil. You can likewise make a straightforward clean by blending 1 cup of olive oil in with 1/4 cup white vinegar. Pour it on a delicate fabric and work it into the wood, cleaning with the grain. Buff till sparkly. Realizing how to clean wood furniture will assist you with keeping your assets looking dazzling, longer.

Chapter 7: Natural floor cleaner disinfectant spray

1. White Vinegar

Produced using acidic corrosive and water, white vinegar is a force cleaner—effectively slicing through oil and evacuating mold, smells, stains, and wax development. On account of its high causticity, white vinegar diminishes surface microscopic organisms, making it a protected choice to dye. In a recent report by the Journal of Environmental Health, vinegar was found to decrease the measure of microscopic organisms on a hard surface, despite the fact that it was less viable than business cleaners. Vinegar will work for the individuals who esteem a sheltered cleaning strategy and need to free their homes of destructive synthetic concoctions, however it won't leave surfaces totally microscopic organisms free.

2. Vodka

Since most vodka is 80 proof, or 40 percent liquor by volume, it tends to be utilized as a disinfectant to expel shape and buildup. Like vinegar, vodka degreases, expels stains, sparkles installations, and invigorates texture—however without the waiting harsh smell. For the most antibacterial force, search for 100-proof vodka (as most locally acquired hand sanitizers contain at any rate 60 percent liquor), and let it sit for a couple of moments so the liquor can carry out its responsibility.

3. Lemon

The citrus extract in lemons works brilliantly on soluble stains like cleanser rubbish found in restrooms and kitchens. Lemons can likewise be utilized to clean non-permeable surfaces and sparkle oxidized metal (clue: use it to make old copper pots and dish shimmer). In a similar report referenced above, lemon likewise attempted to diminish microbes on hard surfaces, yet was less powerful than both vinegar and business cleaners. In spite of the fact that lemon is less successful than vinegar, it surely wins in the aroma division.

4. Hydrogen Peroxide

On the off chance that you at any point got a cut on the play area as a child, you may definitely know the recognizable sting of hydrogen peroxide in real life. Since the 1920s, hydrogen peroxide has been utilized as a germicide on slices in view of its capacities to eliminate microorganisms by separating cell dividers. It can likewise be utilized to murder shape and expel recolors on white dress. Alert ought to be taken when cleaning with hydrogen peroxide, as it will blanch vivid filaments and engraving the outside of stone after some time.

5. Fundamental Oils

Flexible and extraordinary smelling, fundamental oils have a wide scope of therapeutic and recuperating properties. It shocks no one that they are additionally very amazing operators against microorganisms and parasite. When added to vodka or an answer of cleanser and water, some fundamental oils can improve the cleaning properties, freeing your home of shape, buildup, and smelly scents. There are a lot of microscopic organisms battling fundamental oils to browse, especially tea tree, citronella, geranium, lemongrass, orange, and patchouli. At present, researchers are as yet examining fundamental oils' microscopic organisms battling capacities, including its latent capacity use as an anti-microbial.

6. Steam

The basic blend of water and warmth makes for a definitive conservative and synthetic free disinfectant. At the point when warmed to at any rate 200 degrees Fahrenheit, steam not just dispenses with extreme stuck-on stains and oil, yet can likewise disinfect both hard and delicate surfaces. While steaming might be a more slow procedure—at times taking as long as 20 seconds to completely disinfect one region—If utilized appropriately, steam is fit for expelling microorganisms, germs, dust vermin, and different pathogens.

7. Good Mention: Castile Soap

With its underlying foundations in the Castile district of Spain, Castile cleanser, when produced using olive oil, is currently frequently produced using a mix of vegetable oils. Speedy to foam, a drop of Castile cleanser is such's expected to get dishes, baths, or pretty much any surface spotless. While the cleanser for the most part isn't antibacterial all alone, Dr. Bronner's suggests a natively constructed arrangement that adds tea tree basic oil to make your own normally microorganisms battling chemical.